WATER

Water

Michaela Merten

Munich • London

Copyright © 2018 Michaela Merten

German Copyright © Droemer KNAUR Verlag and 2014 by SÜDWEST Verlag.

Originally published in Germany under the title: Water - origin of life

Water

Translated by Annette Charpentier

Edited by Paul Parry

Design by Charlotte Mouncey www.bookstyle.co.uk

Michaela Merten,

81545 Munich, Germany

ISBN 978-3-946547-18-1

Also available as an

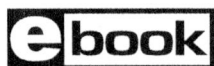

e·book

www.michaela-merten.com
www.happiness-house.de
www.pierre-franckh.com
www.paulparry.com

WATER

the pure truth

Michaela Merten

Contents

PREFACE

Why a book about water?

For the well-being of your body – inside and outside – and your soul, water is the most important element. Water is the source of beauty and health, it heals and balances you. It provides you with energy and makes you wonderfully fit.

Radiant beauty, younger looks, fitness and vitality – water is capable of providing all this for you.

It's so easy: with plenty of water you'll not only reinvigorate yourself but also remain consistently healthy, beautiful and sensual. Drinking plenty of water means being mindful of your body and your soul and giving yourself your full attention.

This book will tell you everything that can be done with the help of water.

I'm looking forward to sharing it with you!

Yours,

Michaela Merten

A short history of water

"Water shows us the way."

LAOTSE

The origins of life

All life originated in the water – and that includes human life as well. Four billion years ago, our planet was surrounded by a toxic layer of ammonium, methane and carbon dioxide, as well as steam. And it was very, very hot. When, eventually, this layer evaporated, our planet cooled. Ultraviolet sun rays triggered the development of a different atmosphere containing mainly hydrogen and carbon dioxide. During a further few million years, the atoms of those two elements realigned themselves, resulting in huge quantities of (water-based) steam, carbon, nitrogen and oxygen.

The vapor came down as rain and gathered in ever-expanding oceans. This process, too, took several million years. During eons of time, all living creatures developed from carbon and water, and only in the water were these microorganisms protected from the lethal rays of the sun. About 450 million years ago, another development began, as the water slowly receded and aquatic creatures had to move on in order to survive. It took millions of years until the first microorganisms and plants dared to become land-based. The first single-cell organisms joined up to become multiple-cellular clusters… and, slowly, the first crawling and flying creatures developed. The first human being probably only evolved about 4 million years ago.

Since the beginning of human development, we have been dependent on the interplay of water and sunshine

It's significant that human blood has the same saline content as sea water: one liter of blood contains 0.9g of salt – evidence that human beings originated in the sea.

The primal oceans have given millions of plants and living creatures their most precious lifeblood – water.

What is water?

Water is a miracle of nature. It has physical properties which, per scientific laws, it shouldn't really have. For example, it expands in a frozen state while other substances shrink. The boiling point of water is about 100 degrees Celsius but, according to the laws of physics, it should be more like minus 46° degrees Celsius. Its highest density is at 4 degrees Celsius – not when it's frozen. Apart from that, water is capable of withstanding the earth's gravity.

Water droplets take the form of spheres, which means that the maximum content is surrounded and held together by the smallest surface. Water is the only substance occurring in three aggregate states: as liquid (water), solid (ice) and gas (steam).

Water is more than the well-known formula of H_2O. This formula symbolises only the two hydrogen atoms and one of oxygen: two hydrogen atoms are grouped around the oxygen atom at an angle of 104.5 degrees.

The French scientist, Antoine Lavoisier, discovered that "the two parts of 'H' – hydrogen – are positively charged and, therefore, electrical, while the one oxygen part – 'O' – tends to be negative and magnetic". Water has a dipolar character. Each molecule contains two electro-magnetic polarities.

When negatively charged electrons are absorbed or discharged, it creates a constantly changing electrical current. Other molecules now can 'dock', meaning that a positively charged H-molecule can randomly join a negative one. Therefore, the molecules are constantly able to join up to create so-called clusters. These clusters can form long chains or join up as networks or bridges.

These hydrogen bridges constantly turn and dance with each other and around each other; they can separate within fractions of a second and rearrange. Their attractive force is so strong that everything in its way will be dissolved or split up. This extraordinary capacity of dissolving matter makes water so important for our body. Our metabolism cannot function at all if we're lacking water – that is, when we don't drink enough.

But water has another fascinating property: it can absorb and transmit information. One assumes the hydrogen bridges to be responsible for this. Because of their crystalline structure the water clusters can store and transmit frequencies of other substances.

Have you ever tried to produce sounds under water? It works! Over vast distances, whales have virtual conversations in the oceans. Ultrasound was developed based on this extraordinary conduciveness. Water is also the most conductive element on the planet.

> Water is not only the 'elixir' of life but also a carrier of signals and messages – negative and positive ones.

Global water circulation

"From outer space our planet is blue"[1] – because 70% of its surface is water. The beauty of our planet is determined by this very special element. An enormous volume of water is constantly shifting. It evaporates, freezes and becomes liquid again, depending on the temperature. Our air contains evaporated water – humidity – and we experience it either as snow, rain or mist. Water evaporates over the oceans, moves towards the coasts as clouds, rains over the hills and mountains before flowing back into the sea.

Water evaporates not only over the oceans but also over land where it rains. Many, many smaller cycles are embedded in the great, overarching cycle of water on earth.

On land, plants absorb most of the water. To maintain photosynthesis and to provide the leafage with nutrients, a forest of, say, four acres, on a warm summer's day, absorbs 40,000 liters of water.

> Hardly anybody knows that only 0.65% of all the water in this world is fresh water

Plants transpire much more water than their own weight. The rest evaporates from the ground, from surface water and habitations. The evaporated water – steam – rises and is cooled down in the higher atmosphere. This cooling down triggers the formation of small droplets, which further condense and form clouds. Depending on the ambient temperature, they fall as rain, snow or hail. But over

1 Heath Robinson, Whale Nation

the oceans much more condensation and evaporation takes place. Nearly 80% of the water evaporating over the oceans also rains there. Only 20% of it is driven by winds towards land to fall there.

Where does "our" water come from?

Our ancestors collected their healthy drinking water from rivers, lakes and springs, enriched with natural oxygen. For modern man, though, this is no longer generally possible because of pollution. Still, we must extract our drinking water from those natural resources. We call it 'raw' or untreated water, because it's taken from a natural source. These sources are:

River water

River water needs to undergo a complicated process to prepare it for human consumption. For that reason, it's often channelled away to seep into the ground where it's cleaned by a natural filtering process. River water is also used as bank filtrate.

Bank filtrate

Here, wells are sunk about 50 to 100 meters away from a river. The river water percolates through the ground towards the wells and is cleansed on its way by earth and rocks. But rivers are often badly polluted and the natural soil filter cannot eliminate all harmful substances.

Groundwater

The hollow parts within the crust of the earth have always been filled with water, and this continues to be the case. These aquifers (reservoirs of water) have developed over centuries of rainfall. Water seeps into the ground and is cleaned and filtered in the process.

Groundwater is still deemed to be the most suitable source of drinking water because it's naturally clean. But as more and more pesticides seep into the ground, its purity is compromised.

Springs

Springs are equally well-suited for the extraction of drinking water. Rising from deep down makes them safe from impurities, but they need protection from pollution and are subject to strict controls imposed by those authorities charged with the springs' well-being. Abstracting drinking water from aquifers and springs is the safest method of obtaining drinking water.

Reservoirs and lakes

Water abstracted from rivers and lakes is called surface water, and needs treatment to achieve drinking-water quality. During one of the treatment processes, acidity is removed, and the water is made sterile through rapid filtering. It's best to abstract the water from the deeper levels of these water bodies, from below 40 meters, because of the lower plankton content.

Mature water

The best water for drinking in my view is so-called 'mature' water – water which has reached the surface in a natural way and without drilling, from deep below the earth's surface, through many layers of rock.

When a porous layer of rock overlays a non-porous one, water which has seeped through from a higher point gathers lower down at the non-porous strata. But the leveling force brings it up to its original level where it springs up.

On its long journey, the water is enriched with natural minerals and filters itself clean. As water always finds its own level and can move upwards in a meandering spiral, it absorbs minerals, filters out impurities and is enriched with energy and information (like its own metadata).

The leveling force of water enables it to rise to a height of up to 2000 meters before reaching the surface, seemingly defying gravity. These springs, flowing freely from deep within the earth, are called *artesian* (after the French region Artois and its particular geological make-up).

This spring water has sometimes been on its way for decades – or even hundreds of years – and is naturally mature. It also has the propensity to purify itself, making it nearly impossible for bacteria to multiply in it. This water can be kept nearly indefinitely because of its strong crystalline structure.

Artesian spring water has a very low surface tension and is very suitable as a cleansing, transporting and dissolving agent for our organisms. It's uniquely suitable for our metabolism and all other physical processes in the human body.

Holy water

Many people all over the globe have honored water as a holy element – and many still do. Every culture, every religion has certain rituals involving water, invoking many different deities. Our fairy stories and old tales feature many fantastic water beings, such as nymphs, river gods, water goddesses, sirens (who drive men crazy), mermaids and selkies.

Churches and other cult sites were often established near a spring, lake or river. Many religions celebrate baptism with water. Often, there was a custom to donate small gifts at the occasion to pacify the water gods and pray that they wouldn't destroy people's homes and goods. The commitment to always give something back for what one has received is a very healthy attitude. That all the elements of heaven and earth relate to each other has always been a powerful guideline – and still is. And because our bodies are part of those elements, everything we do to Mother Nature we also do to ourselves. To revere water has been part of our spiritual and practical heritage since time immemorial.

One of the reasons for water being considered holy is its ability to heal. Each year more than six million pilgrims visit Lourdes in France. The waters in Lourdes seem to have a unique crystalline structure which is capable of triggering the human body's self-healing capacity. Over 600 'miracle cures' in Lourdes have been documented. A miracle cure is acknowledged only when a spontaneous healing continues over several years without the original disease reoccurring.

I mention this because many people dismiss this kind of belief in "miracle cures". But without believing in oneself and one's aims, no building would ever be erected, no invention would get patented, no world record would ever be broken, no progress would be made. Belief is one of the strongest powers in humans. If you don't believe that your health will improve, even the best doctors in the world won't be able to help you.

> Water which has risen on its own, such as in artesian wells, has many vitalizing powers and energies.

Many people have discovered that they find most of their inner strength in the mountains, the forests or by the sea. Watching ocean waves, the ripples of a river or the glittering surface of a lake will always calm our thoughts. In many cultures the immersion in water equals a cleansing of the soul. Once you acknowledge the power of water, you'll realize very soon its beneficial effects in every way.

Did you know...?

- More than 71% of the earth's surface is covered by salt water.

- Only 0.65% of the whole body of water on the planet is fresh or 'sweet' water.

- Water reserves on earth don't decrease but must be shared between more and more people.

- Every year the world's population grows by 80 million people, adding to the current 7.2 billion – that is a daily increase of 233,280 people.

- Individuals' water consumption rises constantly. On average, we use about 122 liters per day, of which only 2 liters are for drinking.

- Hotels on average use 350 liters of water a day per guest, golf hotels up to 800 liters per day.

- Pesticides, heavy metals and slurry used by agriculture pollute rivers and lakes. Toxic substances seep through the soil into the groundwater. Decades of mankind's unrestricted use of pollutants have had a dramatic effect on our groundwater today.

One liter of rainwater absorbs the contaminants of 350,000 liters of air (acid rain).

Our drinking water contains up to 700 substances reacting with each other – which so far have not been researched.

Agriculture is the biggest end-user of water.

In drought periods, all required water needs to be taken from rivers and lakes. Around the globe, about 70% of fresh water is extracted this way.

To produce a kilogram of grain, 1,500 liters of water is needed. A kilogram of citrus fruit needs 1,000 liters to grow. It takes 15,000 liters of water to produce a kilogram of beef.

It takes around 400,000l of water to paint and finish a car.

1.2 billion people don't have any access to clean fresh water. 2.5 billion – about a third of the world's population – have no access to a sewage system.

Each year, five million people perish because of polluted water; every day, 6,000 children die because of a lack of clean water.

At the time of writing, 14 countries don't have sufficient water reserves for their population.

The United Nations has stated that another nine countries will join this group by 2025.

A lack of sewage systems, in combination with polluted drinking water, are – according to UNESCO – the main reasons (80%) for diseases in developing countries.

Future wars will be fought for the control of water. Access to and control of rivers, lakes and the sea will be hotly contested. 261 rivers around the globe cross borders.

*

The water in our body

"Every raindrop is a kiss from heaven."
FRIEDENSREICH HUNDERTWASSER (1928-2000),
AUSTRIAN ARTIST

Water, the elixir of life

We are creatures of water. From birth until death, our body needs water in the same way as it requires oxygen and food. For the first nine months of our lives we're actually completely immersed in water – but we don't remember that. Water makes up 70% of our bodies, and an even higher proportion of our brains

Many indigenous people worship water as a holy element. All alternative healing programs make us aware of how precious this primal element is and utilize it for healing purposes. Today, in mainstream society, the healing powers of water have been largely forgotten – but water is the most important element in our lives.

As soon as we don't take in enough water, the body switches into an emergency mode and prioritizes its reserves. The brain is the first to be supplied with the necessary fluids before the main organs. If this happens, the rest of the body not only suffers because of those priorities but its own reserves are used too. And as soon as the water level in body cells drops, many functions and metabolic processes slow down or are reduced. During a phase of decreasing water levels in the body we receive subtle signals – but we mostly ignore them. We may notice the first slight impairments, such as headaches, dry eyes, a lack of concentration. Then we often quickly just take a pill in the belief that all will be well. But this is the wrong step – and it could have dire consequences for your body.

Everybody knows that plants die when they don't get enough water. Why should we be less important than a plant? We don't get the life-giving liquid in the form of rain, mist or by a watering can, so we have no other choice than to drink it. The minimum amount is two liters of water a day, which should not be drunk in one go, but consumed over the day. The biorhythm and functions of our body need a constant supply of water. Water is the medium for transporting and dissolving matter around the body, as well as for filtering and cleansing. It's vital for every process within our body. It's not good enough when, after not drinking much during the day, we remember it in the evening and try to make up for it by swallowing it in large gulps. Our body works every second of the day. The blood, with its high water content, transports nutrients, oxygen and pollutants within the body or discharges them. Without sufficient water, pollutants cannot be filtered out by the kidneys and the liver, but these toxins need to go somewhere. Without enough water, we create a kind of 'retoxification', because the toxins will be deposited elsewhere in the body.

> With a sufficient water intake, you can reduce the risk of contracting an illness by up to 70%. By drinking enough water, we activate our self-healing powers and the whole metabolism is activated and boosted.

It's important to learn – again – to listen to our body. It constantly sends us messages. But we have forgotten to understand its language. The body is able to inform us about deficiences only by a feeling of unease and, eventually, pain and illness. When we numb this pain without thoroughly trying to explore its causes, we quickly fall into a negative cycle which is very difficult to break.

Unfortunately, there is a common belief that we take in enough liquid by drinking coffee, tea or soft drinks. This is a grave error, because those drinks give us a sense of quenching the thirst, but for the body this causes exactly the opposite: in fact, those drinks dehydrate, they draw water from the body to leave it in a state of chronic dehydration.

Older people are particularly affected by this. With age, the sense of thirst weakens, often with bad consequences: memory issues, joint problems, backaches – all this can be the result of a chronic lack of hydration.

Water is not only our number one food, it's also our best cosmetic aid. The human skin needs a lot of moisture, and when this is lacking, it develops wrinkles and loses its elasticity. We evaporate half a liter of water a day through the skin, and even more when exercising. The wrinkling process can only partly be remedied by expensive moisturizers. The best cosmetic aid is still just water. Skin cells can only be plump and smooth when they get enough moisture. It's indispensable for a smooth skin – and so easy – to feed it moisture from within in the form of water.

Drink, drink, drink... but only water

Each day, take in at least two liters of water. When exercising, especially in the warmer months, even more.

Water is life-preserving...

... for your cells

Water is the most important transport agent within our organism. It brings oxygen to every single cell, collects the detritus and transports it to the lungs to be exhaled. Approximately 13 billion cells in our body are embedded in water, and in those cells all substances entering the body are transformed and assimilated.

... for your joints

Lubricants within the joints diminish with age, which can lead to arthritis and backaches. One signal for a general lack of water can be joint pains, the worst-case scenario being that the bones might rub against each other without any cushioning. Apart from stabbing pains, this can cause rheumatism and other inflammations. With enough water the body's joints remain supple, and general suppleness isn't just a pleasant feeling but also a sign of youthfulness.

Only with the help of water can the discs in our spine act as efficient buffers between the vertebrae. These discs are working hard day in, day out. All the time they cushion blows and jolts when we're walking, running or jumping. The discs consist of nearly 85% water and can function properly as our inner springs only when they're properly hydrated. To perform perfectly and without pain they need a constant supply of water.

... for your skin

Of course, we all get older, but that doesn't mean that we should look it. Your skin needs water badly; without a sufficient supply your skin practically dries out. The lack of water can only partly be remedied by expensive moisturizers because the skin needs fluids from within.

> TIP: for maintaining beautiful skin, healthy looks and a positive attitude, we need to re-learn to listen to our body. That way, we regain our natural balance and can skip through life.

When the body's interior is drying out, your skin cells practically shrink, and they can blossom and shine only when they get what they need – water.

... for your blood

Water thins the blood. This lessens the risk of a stroke or blood clotting. With sufficient water the blood pressure can decrease. If the water content of your blood falls, it can result in lethargy and difficulties concentrating.

Our blood, in an optimal and well-supplied state, consists of nearly 94% water.

We should drink water, constantly, day after day, so that there is always enough blood circulating around our body.

... for your lungs

Red blood cells can store oxygen only when they're sufficiently saturated. With every breath, we evaporate water. Alveoli – the tiny air bubbles within the lungs – are very sensitive and need to be constantly supplied with an adequate amount of water to function properly. If that's not the case, when they're not sufficiently plumped up, the bronchioles, the 'branches' of alveoli, become more susceptible to illness. Every day we lose about 1.2 liters of water by breathing and through the skin and, of course, much more when exercising.

... for your genes

Water can prevent damage to the genetic equipment. The process of repairing DNA is well supported by water.

... for your heart

Our heart is a two-way pump, sucking blood in and pumping it out. Just as water in our natural environment, blood moves in a meandering way through the whole organism.

As a sufficient supply of water in the body can lower the blood pressure, the heart needs to work less, which can help to prevent a heart attack. Conversely, when the body loses more than 10% of its water content, we're more likely to suffer a stroke or a heart attack.

> When the body loses more than 20% of its liquids the organism enters a life-threatening state.

... for your kidneys and liver

Water supports the functions of the most important detoxifying organs of the body. It flushes out toxins and dissolves harmful deposits. If, because of a lack of water, those organs can't function properly, the body suffers a kind of 're-toxification'. The kidneys filter and cleanse the equivalent of about 180 liters of liquids every day. About two liters are discarded in the form of urine. If your urine has a pale colour and is clear, you drink enough water. A darker, brownish coloration indicates dehydration.

... for your brain

Headaches, tiredness, memory loss and a lack of concentration are only a few of the symptoms of a brain that's not sufficiently hydrated. Consisting of about 95% water, the brain virtually swims in its own 'water bed', known as 'brain fluid'. If not sufficiently supplied with water, the brain very quickly sends out pain signals. The brain is also involved in the production of hormones. Day by day, the equivalent of about 1,400 liters of blood pass through our brain.

... for connective tissue

Connective tissue has an important function for the whole body. It can store a lot of water as its cells are able to absorb fluids like a sponge. When connective tissue is constantly supplied with enough water, it remains firm and elastic.

... for your eyes

The eye consists of nearly 99% water. Due to polluted air, a lack of oxygen or too much screen work, they can dry out. Drinking lots of water prevents this unpleasant symptom. Tears are made up of water and salt. We need this liquid to constantly moisten the eyeball. Well-moistened, clear eyes are regarded as a sign of beauty and enhance people's attractiveness.

... for your bones

Our bones, apparently so hard and solid, still contain about 22% water. With insufficient quantities of water, the body reacts by gathering the reserves from other places, including bones. One result can be brittle bones (osteoporosis). The increasing risk of fractures in older people, often caused by osteoporosis, can be reduced by drinking enough water.

...for your muscles

Eating good quality fruit and vegetables is a good way to keep your muscles strong.

Well-exercised muscles contain up to 75% water. To keep our muscles strong and supple, the body needs a lot of water.

Well-formed muscles contribute to a well-shaped, beautiful body.

... for the metabolism

Nearly all metabolic processes are initiated by water, which is the most important medium for transporting and dissolving nutrients and toxins. There are many signs indicating a lack of water in the body. Maybe you have simply forgotten to interpret those signals. We generally believe that a dry mouth is the first sign of feeling thirsty, but that's not the case. The first signs of thirst can be heartburn, a lack of concentration, hunger, headaches, neck aches, irritability, halitosis, joint pains, pains when walking or a low mood. Many, many symptoms can indicate a single cause: that we're not drinking enough – or we're drinking the wrong stuff.

> TIP: don't wait until you feel thirsty – just develop a habit of drinking two liters of water every day. Put a couple of liter bottles of water and a glass near you, on your desk perhaps, and keep drinking small quantities all day until both bottles are empty. For every cup of coffee, which dehydrates, you should drink two glasses of water. That way the kidneys get a chance to detoxify and flush out the caffeine. Actually, it's much better to replace coffee with unsweetened herbal teas. Commercially produced fruit juices and lemonades are no healthy alternative as they often contain artificial sweeteners which can be harmful for the enzymes in our body.

Water enhances your beauty

Water can give you a youthful look. Young people everywhere fascinate and attract because they seem to radiate from inside and move in a supple, graceful way. How can you preserve those signs of youthfulness?

A very important step towards this is certainly a sensible diet. And the main part? Water. You'll notice it very quickly: if you change your normal habits and start drinking two liters of water a day, you'll immediately feel more alive and energetic. Your skin will soon start to radiate as if from an inner light.

The skin is our largest organ, with about two square meters of surface. Day and night, it works very hard, and it's most perfectly organized. A virtual army of cells, all with specific functions, ensures that all its tasks are carried out most accurately.

Every day the skin evaporates nearly two liters of water in the form of sweat – and, of course, more when exercising. This loss of fluid needs to be replenished. Beautiful skin is smooth and elastic. As soon as skin cells are given the opportunity to soak up enough water, the skin becomes smoother from inside out.

How much water do we need?

As our body can't store the water we need day in, day out, we should constantly supply it with the precious liquid. Close your eyes and imagine the following: you are an aquarium in your living room and you daily lose a certain amount of water by evaporation. If it's hot outside, even more water disappears. If you own an aquarium you'll know that you need to replenish the water daily so that the creatures living in it won't die.

Your body organs and metabolic processes are equally happy when they regularly receive enough water to go on living. As the human body loses a relatively high amount of water over 24 hours, this loss needs to be replenished by continuously drinking water.

The formula for a sufficient supply of drinking water is your bodyweight in kilograms x 0.30. For a person of, say, 65kg, this means 65 x 0.30 = 1.95 litres. This person needs to drink about two liters of water per day, and increase the amount when exercising.

Nothing can replace water

We will now look at a widely-believed error that alcohol, coffee, tea and soft drinks give us enough liquids during the day. Those drinks certainly contain a large amount of water, as they're water-based, but the added ingredients and substances diminish its effect as they virtually flush water from the body. And there is worse to come: those drinks cost your organism additional water and they deplete its precious reserves even more.

> TIP: you should drink 30ml of water per kg of your bodyweight each day.

The daily habit of drinking coffee, tea and other drinks containing caffeine, plus maybe a glass or two of beer or other alcoholic drink, can cause dire consequences within your body. Even though you're drinking a lot of liquids, you're gradually drying out inside.

The nasty feeling of a hangover after a long boozy night means that your brain has been depleted of water. As the brain reacts particularly sensitively to a lack of water, it's practically crying for it in that state.

But not just your brain is at risk of damage due to the wrong kind of drinks – our most important digestive organ, the gut, is placed under stress, too. Our gut, because of years spent dealing with an unsuitable diet containing refined sugar (which has a paralyzing effect on this organ), is now less able to produce all the enzymes required for processing food. Here, too, the consequences can be clearly felt because our immune system becomes vulnerable.

> TIP: drink water! Nothing can replace water. And if you feel like drinking tea, then choose herbal or fruit tea. There is a great variety of delicious teas on offer. Try to sweeten it with honey like our ancestors. Honey is a more intense sweetener than sugar and you don't need as much - which is good for the weight...

One way of breaking this negative cycle would be a cleansing of the gut – either by colonic irrigation or several days of fasting, followed by a change of diet. A good start for this kind of inner rejuvenation is to adopt the habit of constantly replenishing your inner water table. This will give your whole body the chance to deal with pollutants and toxins.

The blood-brain barrier in infants and young children

The human brain has a very effective mechanism to protect itself from the varying composition of the body's blood and possible toxins contained in it: the blood-brain barrier.

The brain needs a lot of energy. The tiny blood vessels inside the brain are called capillaries – and there are about 640km

The blood-brain barrier isn't completely developed in babies and toddlers, which makes it extremely important to give them only the purest and best food and water.

of them in this organ alone, with a surface of nine square meters! These blood vessels are minute and, unlike normal blood vessels, nearly impenetrable.

A very effective filtering system prevents harmful substances such as nicotine, alcohol, proteins and non-soluble fats from entering the brain.

The barrier works in two ways. First of all, glial cells – non-neuronal cells that provide support and protection for neurons in the central and peripheral nervous systems surrounding the blood vessels and help us maintain balance – prevent the penetration of non-soluble fats and proteins. Only the exchange of ions and other simple molecular substances is permitted. As well as that, endothelin cells act as a filter, as they constrict blood vessels and raise blood pressure.

Before the blood-brain barrier is fully developed, as with infants and small children, or when it's damaged by other factors or harmful substances entering the brain, it can result in neurological damage. Should those substances settle within the brain, they can damage it over time.

Dr Leif Salford, of the Lund University in Sweden, is a renowned neurologist. For decades, he's been researching changes in the blood-brain barrier.

"Their results have been consistent and alarming: not only does radiation from a cell phone damage the blood-brain barrier, but it does so even when the exposure level is reduced a thousand-fold. Even more disturbingly, and contrary to what was expected, the damage to the blood-brain barrier worsened when the experimenters reduced the exposure level. The implies that SAR [specific absorption rate] ratings for cell phones may be worthless and that it may not be possible to make cell phones safer by reducing their power.

In laboratory rats, Salford's team has demonstrated that blood-brain barrier leakage occurs after only two minutes of exposure. Further, a single two-hour exposure to a cell phone, even at reduced power, was shown to damage or destroy up to 2% of an animal's brain cells.

In other experiments in Salford's laboratory, long-term exposure of rats to a cell phone caused memory impairment, and a single six-hour exposure at extremely low-power levels caused genetic damage. Exposure to a low-frequency magnetic field (low frequencies are also emitted by cell phones) caused disturbances of calcium transport in cells.

Salford has called the use of cell phones by human beings "the largest biological experiment ever", and he calls the potential implications of his laboratory results "terrifying". "Those who might normally have got Alzheimer's dementia in old age could get it much earlier," he said. "Perhaps putting a mobile phone repeatedly to your head is something that might not be good in the long term."[2]

*

In the production of baby food, one needs to observe even stricter levels of purity. Firstly, any water used needs to be low in natrium. If mineral water is used, there are certain upper limits of substances contained in it:

Nitrate – below 10milligrams per liter (mg/l)

Nitrite – below 0.02mg/l

Natrium – below 20mg/l

Sulphate – below 240mg/l (the lower the better)

Fluoride – below 1.5mg/l (I recommend we stay well below the suggested upper limit, as most toothpastes and some bread already contain a certain amount of fluoride)

2 http://www.cellphonetaskforce.org/?page_id=579

Colonic hydrotherapy

In recent years, death rates through colonic cancer have risen sharply. The colon (the whole intestine, including large and small) is our most important digestive organ, with a surface of 32 square meters and between 5.5 and 7.5 meters in length!

More than 80% of the immune system is located in the gut. This makes it one of the most important organs for our overall health.

Within the small and the large intestine our food is separated into digestible and non-digestible parts. The indigestible matter is excreted and the important nutrients transported to the rest of the body.

A healthy gut prevents pathogenic (harmful) substances from entering the rest of the body, and a healthy mucus membrane within the gut is indispensable for a functioning immune system. But life today can expose us to almost constant physical stress. Our digestive system is extremely challenged by a bad diet, lack of water, too much coffee and nicotine and by eating too quickly, so even a healthy bacterial environment in the gut is constantly compromised. This could result in constipation, allergies and a variety of illnesses.

There is an effective method to expel environmental toxins from the body – and it's also based on the cleansing powers of water: colonic hydrotherapy– a kind of enema which is best performed by a natural-health practitioner or a doctor. In this procedure, water of body temperature is inserted into the gut, while at the same time the stomach is massaged to loosen up possible rigidifications.

Following years of consuming a poor diet and processed food, the villi in the gut – small protrusions which separate nutrients from waste and absorb them – are hopelessly clogged up. The whole system is overwhelmed and no longer capable of ejecting all the waste products. And when the villi are clogged up or blocked, the nutrients your body needs can't be absorbed anymore even if your diet is healthy. The gut slows down and doesn't move like it should, which results in a much more prolonged digestive process. Constipation ensues, while the body signals its need for nutrients.

And you continue with your healthy diet and wonder why you put on weight!

Being overweight and suffering from malnutrition – it's a paradox. You can save all the money you might want to spend on laxatives – just have your gut cleansed professionally and thoroughly. Once is enough. Sometimes, during a colonic irrigation, sediments which have clogged up your guts for up to 20 years are removed. Many people, a lot of them suffering from allergies and migraine, benefit tremendously from colonic hydrotherapy.

Please attend to this hard-working organ from time to time. Be kind to it and help it to get moving again. You need it…

The best drinking water

Clean water for a healthy body

As far back as the 1950s, the French hydrologist Louis Claude Vincent published a study pointing out the correlation between the quality of drinking water and death and sickness rates. For decades now our environment has been showered with pesticides, herbicides and fungicides – and it continues. The harmful effect of this has become so evident that nobody can deny it anymore. Agricultural fields in Germany alone are covered with about 35,000 tons of pesticides, slurry and artificial manure every year. With rain, these substances filter into the groundwater. In addition, air pollutants are also brought down to ground-level by rain. We simply need to develop more awareness that all those toxic substances are very detrimental for the human body and cause numerous illnesses.

> TIP: if you wish to improve the quality of your tap water, do some research on water filters and purifying devices. There are numerous ways to cleanse your drinking water for personal use.

For the human body, it's vitally important to drink only clear, pure and revitalizing water. During the eons of our development as human beings, our body hasn't changed much, and it can't find this vital source of life in any other foodstuff. Soft drinks, sugared fruit juice and – even worse – drinks with artificial sweeteners wreak havoc with your metabolism. The results are obesity and many illnesses which are also caused by malnutrition.

Our drinking water

Let's have a look at the water we use day in, day out in our homes, water we use to meet our daily needs: tap water. It's water we have access to 24 hours a day. It's pure enough for us to drink but we use 98% of it for domestic cleaning! Depending on our needs, it's delivered to us hot, warm and cold and, until recently, we have hardly given this fact any attention.

Luckily there are more and more people now debating the role of our drinking water. Health aspects have entered the discussion, as we slowly develop awareness that it's the individual who should take responsibility for his or her wellbeing. The best start for this process is to begin where everything has begun: with the purity of our water.

The good news is that the water companies guarantee the drinking water quality of our tap water. The less good news is that most of the substances in our drinking water are not being considered by the water companies. Tap water needs to be "free from any micro-organisms and parasites and from any substances which, in numbers or concentrations, constitute a potential danger to human health", it says in the European Drinking Water Directive.

Tap water of drinking quality has been taken for granted for a very long time, and it's difficult to better appreciate this precious commodity.

The law sees to it that there are no germs and viruses in our drinking water with the potential to cause widespread illness. Bacteria, fungi, viruses and other germs are filtered out in the complex treatment process carried out by the water companies. Many substances aren't being filtered out, but the directive gives clear upper limits for some.

TIP: ask your local water company where your drinking water originates. Then you still can decide whether to install a filtering system in your house. As you drink only about 2% of the tap water, it might be a consideration to replace tap water for your personal use by high quality mineral water. What could be damaging to an infant could also damage you over the years. You want to avoid environmental toxins as much as you can.

But if a substance is not mentioned in the directive, it doesn't have to be filtered out. For that reason, babies and toddlers should never be given tap water for drinking, nor should their meals be prepared with it.

The quality of tap water differs from region to region. It's said that the water Londoners drink has gone through them fourteen times before. Some areas extract drinking water from deep groundwater levels and it has undergone a natural cleansing process. Other areas gain their tap water from surface waters but, should those areas be near roads with heavy traffic or an industrial district, the water is polluted by environmental toxins.

Upper limits

In many areas, water companies aim to produce a product that's within the official upper limits of impurities. You'll have probably heard about the many different opinions of scientists and politicians regarding drinking water. But the European directive sets the upper limits for the whole Union so Europeans can rely on the cleanliness of their tap water.

But it remains a difficult subject, because even with so many restrictions there are lots of substances which aren't even listed on the directive. Residues of medication or hormones are neither considered nor on anybody's list so far.

Aluminum, for example, is suspected to contribute to the development of dementia or Alzheimer's disease. The European upper limit for infants is set at 0.2mg per liter. Young children, infants, sick and old people are particularly susceptible to environmental toxins, but who knows whether you yourself might not be susceptible? Do you know which particular substances you react negatively to? Are you satisfied that the upper limits of your tap water's toxic substances are acceptable for your body?

These upper limits indicate that governments accept noxious substances in our drinking water, but only in quantities intended to avoid illness for those consuming it. But who knows which limits are the right ones for you?

Noxious substances

These, clearly, are substances which damage our body. A healthy body has an incredible capacity to regenerate and heal, but we shouldn't make these tasks unnecessarily difficult by consuming heavy metals (ie, metals such as lead and copper, which have a high density) and medication we don't need.

Year in, year out we bombard our body with noxious substances present in the food that we eat. In addition, we take hormones, such as contraceptive pills and, by excreting them, residues enter the water system. This is not reflected in the regulations regarding drinking water, and it would be difficult to assess and eliminate those residues.

Noxious substances within our body can accumulate to dangerous levels. Add the pollutants in the environment, our homes and radiating from electronic devices– and it becomes an obligation to pay good attention to what you eat and drink every day. Yes, we know that our drinking water has to be free from contaminants and germs, but in the end it's you who decides what kind of water you drink.

> Everybody has a different diet and takes in, every day, varying additional harmful substances in both their drinking water and food.

The list of known harmful substances and their upper limits implies that, even when ingested for a lifetime, they're not damaging. But don't rely on regulations like this. Instead, take control of what you eat and drink.

> Nitrates are present in higher concentration in areas dominated by agriculture. In the human body, nitrates turn into *nitrites*, and nitrites attach to red blood cells, which suffer as a consequence and can't properly perform their task of carrying oxygen to the body's cells. This can result in a lack of oxygen in the whole body.

> The presence of chlorine and chlorine dioxide are, equally, reasons to be careful. They're supposed to kill off germs, but chlorine and chlorides tend to bond with other substances.

> The presence of medication residues in drinking water can't be eradicated by even the best filtering systems. They return, time and again, to the drinking water cycle.

Water pipes

Pollution of your drinking water increases on the water's long journey to your tap. Water companies today acknowledge the fact that drinking water, as it travels way to people's homes, can change and be polluted by additional harmful substances.

If you live in an old house or a flat with water pipes made from lead, it could be that your water has a lead content way above the legal upper limit – which in fact is zero. Lead was used for drinking-water pipes up to the Seventies. The symptoms of lead poisoning due to lead water pipes are chronic tiredness, apathy or lack of drive. Lead is a toxin which attacks the nervous system, and is poisonous even in very small quantities.

Traces of copper, too, are often found in drinking water. Tap water pipes made from lead, copper and other metals continuously feed tiny particles into the water. Another problem is caused by the length of time water remains in the pipe because, often, several hours pass between openings of the tap. In most cases, regulations for drinking water are valid at the point of exit from the treatment plant, not at the tap.

Water has a very high capacity to dissolve, and this is detrimental where pipes are concerned, as they have a layer within them to protect from corrosion, but who knows the exact details of their home's construction?

The hardness or softness of drinking water is also important. If the water contains too much calcium and magnesium ions they can form deposits in the pipes and electric kettles. To reduce water's calcium content, chlorine or chlorine dioxide is added.

Asbestos fibers, too, often get into drinking water, as pipes made of the material being used until 1990 are now slowly deteriorating. Such substances and heavy metals are primarily deposited in the brain, bones and gut.

Interdependency

We now know that not all harmful substances are listed in drinking-water regulations. The several thousand tonnes of pesticides, herbicides and fungicides that are spread on fields annually across the world for agricultural purposes enter the food chain, too. These toxins seep into the ground and eventually get into the groundwater. That is one reason to dig deeper and deeper to abstract clean drinking water, but because of the sheer volume of water extracted for drinking purposes, the groundwater level is sinking, and the water has no time to clean itself through filtering.

All these potentially harmful substances in our drinking water can react with each other in a way so-far unknown.

Residues of medication enter the water through human excretion. Year after year, medication which is past its sell-by date is also tipped into the sewage system. The same is true of birth-control pills. Additionally, there are numerous microorganisms in this toxic cocktail, as well as waste products from chlorine. Scientists don't know yet whether the elements of this evil concoction react with each other with very negative consequences. All those substances can bond with each other, form clusters and maybe damage the human body.

Pressure in the pipes

Only in recent years has the natural flowing capacity of water become a topic of discussion. Water molecules (known as clusters) form chains, networks and bridges. The basic character of water is that it moves in a spiraling way. But if water is forced, by pressure, to flow through narrow pipes, it loses its natural flowing capacity.

In the northern hemisphere, water moves in a spiraling, meandering way, clockwise. This meandering movement creates levitant forces which enable water to rise from very deep down in the earth and thus provide us with spring water. Because of a pressure of roughly

Alternative water scientists and nature observers have been researching *dead* and *alive* water for decades, but modern mainstream science doesn't acknowledge this.

6 bar – and the long journey through the pipes – water loses its natural structure. The change in the liquid's structure becomes measurable after an 80-meter-journey through a pipe. The clusters are compressed and get lumpy. Our drinking water becomes 'dead' water, which needs to be brought back to its original form to be of vital importance to the human body.

Turning right or turning left?

In the northern hemisphere, fresh spring water turns clockwise, to the right. In the southern hemisphere – in Australia, for example – the spiral turns counterclockwise, to the left.

You might have observed this phenomenon: if you drain the water from a bath, it flows down in a spiraling way.

> "At the end of the century, a liter of water will be dearer than a liter of wine."
>
> VICTOR SCHAUBERGER, 1935

Mineral waters

There are numerous brands of mineral water on the market, some of which have been declared as healing and particularly pure. Many countries produce their own brand, their own bottled healing spring water. This creates quite a lot of confusion about which water is best to drink.

> TIP: you can return the natural flowing behavior to your 'dead' water by pouring it through a funnel or installing a special device to the tap which influences the direction of the water flow.

Bottled water

Bottled water, like tap water, is subject to strict regulations. There are special regulations for water claiming healing properties.

Natural mineral water

This kind of water is subject to special conditions. It has to originate from aquifers underground which are protected from pollution and other impurities. It naturally contains minerals and trace elements. It can be obtained from different springs, is constantly controlled and bottled at source.

In most cases, it contains natural carbon dioxide, it sparkles. It can be enriched with additional carbon. Sometimes the label claims that it is 'de-ironed', meaning that iron is extracted, because it can color the water and influence the taste. Sulphur, too, is extracted from bottled spring water.

Despite a European directive, some imported mineral waters have higher upper limits of potentially harmful substances. Not all ingredients have to be declared.

Spring water

Spring water originates in deep groundwater reservoirs and is also bottled at source. It doesn't have to be completely pure, but must meet all the criteria for drinking water.

It's bottled and sold without further procedures and can come from natural as well as artificially drilled sources. It doesn't need an official certificate.

Mineral water with less than 5.5g carbonic acid is called still mineral water. It also needs to be officially certified.

Table water

Table water can be a mixture of different kinds of water or be just tap water, enriched with minerals and carbonated. Sometimes seawater, salt or oxygen are added.

Table water can be prepared and bottled anywhere, but the labeling shouldn't contain a place name or spring reference. The word 'natural' on the label is not allowed.

Spa water

This kind of water is a freely available medication, a natural water which has found its way from aquifers below, well protected from impurities and containing natural minerals. It's bottled at source. In earlier times, it gave rise to spas, such as Bath, where people went for a cure, "taking" the waters. Today, it can be bought bottled.

Depending on the area, it will have filtered through several layers of rock and is suitable for various complaints and illnesses. Healing water from springs is naturally pure. It's more expensive than other bottled water because its efficacy has been tried and tested in various procedures. The healing, preventative or soothing characteristics will have been officially confirmed.

Oxygenated water

This kind of water has become quite fashionable. It's enriched with oxygen, like nature intended, because spring water always contains oxygen. But the human body is only capable of taking in oxygen via breathing and the lungs, not via the gut. Sometimes oxygenated water contains more than 20 times the normal oxygen in spring water. Even normal tap water can be enriched and sold as oxygenated water.

The minerals in mineral water

This is another hotly debated question, like the upper limits for drinking water. Natural mineral water contains minerals and trace elements. This is how it reaches the surface after traveling from deep down in the earth. But it doesn't only contain 'good' substances, but also 'bad' ones, such as heavy metals and nitrates.

We already obtain enough minerals and trace elements with our diet – as long the diet is balanced. Apart from that, the minerals dissolved in the mineral water can't be easily absorbed by the human body.

The human body can process only 5% of minerals in the water we drink

You might as well suck on a pebble in the belief you would ingest some healthy minerals. The minerals in drinking water are inorganic and hardly digestible for the human body. We're able to digest organic minerals from only plants.

Chemically speaking, organic and inorganic minerals are the same, but not for the human body which needs minerals in a different form.

The minerals plants absorb from the environment through their leaves and roots are optimally digestible for our body.

Inorganic minerals, which dissolve in only water, aren't able to react in the body for metabolic purposes. The best examples are calcium and iron: both substances need to be adapted by the stomach's acid to our metabolism. If you don't have enough stomach acid, those minerals circulate in the body in their original form and can settle in joints and blood vessels. The same applies to mineral pills.

Plastic bottle or glass bottle?

This is another hot topic: the plastic bottle. Of course, it's more comfortable, simpler and lighter to transport water in plastic bottles. But compared with glass bottles they have significant disadvantages. Remember, water molecules are constantly moving…

In a glass bottle, water molecules move naturally because they can push against the harder glass wall to rotate. With a plastic bottle, it's different. Between the plastic layer and the water molecules a kind of vacuum forms which cannot push the water molecules hard enough to turn and rotate. They don't move naturally and lose their vitality – and kind of run out of steam. Water in plastic bottles has lost its vitality and energy.

Water is also a carrier of information and can adopt the taste of plastic. Glass is an organic material and most suitable for keeping and transporting drinking water.

You can try this out yourself. Put a plastic bottle filled with water into the fridge next to a cut-up melon. After two days, the water tastes of melon.

Earlier generations used carafes and drinking glasses made from rock crystal to contain the precious stuff. If the water takes in the crystal-clear information, you can only wonder how our ancestors had obtained this important knowledge. Nobody at that time had done any research on the molecular structure of water…

Minerals and trace elements

Please have a close look at the label of your favorite mineral water. In the following, I explain the various substances and abbreviations so you understand more clearly what you're putting into your body.

pH = the concentration of the hydrogen ions (expressing acidity and alkalinity)

You'll have heard of the so-called pH value. Regarding mineral water, it means that the water should be as neutral as possible with a pH value of around 6.8 or 6.9. Drinks with a pH value lower than 7 are acidic. And, as our organism is chronically too acidic anyway, please observe the balance between alkaline and acidic.

Soluble substances

This indicates how many trace elements and minerals are contained in one liter of water. It's calculated by condensing the water and measuring the residual substances.

Aluminum (Al) You probably know the light metal aluminum from various household products. You can find it in drinks cans, yoghurt pot lids, cake

mixtures and other products. For the past few years there has been a debate whether aluminum might contribute to the development of Alzheimer's disease. The World Health Organization denied this claim in 1997. Aluminum doesn't present a risk to people unless they're constantly confronted with it at work. But it's proven that too much aluminum can trigger stomach and gut problems and cause a lack of energy, speech difficulties and senility. The aluminum content in drinking water should stay below 0.01 milligrams per liter (mg/l), but drinking water regulations state twice this amount is permissible. In addition, we take in more aluminum with our food.

Arsenic (As) A certain dose of arsenic is lethal for the human body, but many mineral waters contain traces of arsenic, but well below the upper limit of 10 nanograms per liter (ng/l). Imported mineral waters might have different upper limits. When preparing baby food particularly, you should see that there is no arsenic in the water, not even traces. If you follow homoeopathic rules you would avoid mineral waters with traces of arsenic anyway. Even the tiniest amounts can cause nausea, dizziness, damage to the blood vessels and a decrease in the production of red blood cells. Some studies have stated a correlation between arsenic and cancer. Scientists and drinking water regulations recommend an arsenic content below 0.01mg/l. For table water, it can be as high as 0.05mg/l.

Calcium (Ca) Calcium is the main mineral building-block for our bones. A continuous lack of calcium often results in age-related osteoporosis and can increase the risk of a heart attack. The heart, the nerves and the muscles need calcium. The calcium contained in cow's milk can't be digested by the human body sufficiently – quite the opposite: it struggles with it. Too much calcium can cause a lack of appetite and constipation.

Carbon dioxide (Co2) Carbon dioxide is a non-toxic gas. It's colorless and hardly has a smell. It occurs naturally in mineral water or can be added to it, making it sparkling. Carbon dioxide is also used in the sewage industry to keep water clean. When you drink alcohol in combination with carbonated water, it increases the speed of alcohol absorption in the brain.

Chlorine (Cl) We all know chlorine as a disinfective agent for swimming pools. In some areas chlorine is added to the drinking water as well. Chlorine and natrium are the components of our cooking salt. The transport of clean drinking water over ever-growing distances results in the additional problem of bacterial contamination in the pipes which needs to be treated with sterilizing substances. Additional chlorine often binds with other substances and can form trichloroethane, which is suspected to cause colon and bladder cancer. Following the addition of chlorine to drinking water in the US, in 1921, there was a drastic increase in leg problems (about 500%). Drinking water regulations set an upper limit of 250 mg/l.

Copper (Cu) Just like iron, copper is a vital element for the human body. It helps the formation of red blood cells. A lack of copper can contribute to heart disease and reduce tension in the blood vessels. Too much copper – maybe because the pipes for your drinking water contain copper – can cause liver damage. Amalgamate, used in dentistry, can also contain copper. The upper limit for drinking water is 2.0 mg/l.

Chromium (Cr) Chromium is a trace element and important for glucose metabolism. Too much chromium damages mucus membranes and can lead to stomach and colon inflammation as well as liver and kidney damage. Heavy metals get into the environment by refuse incineration and via the sewage system and can be an increasing risk for the human body. In small doses chromium is important for the metabolism of carbs. The upper limit in drinking water regulations is 50ng/l.

Fluoride (F) Fluoride is a necessary building-block for bones and teeth. Toothpastes regularly contain fluoride, which is the reason to be careful with additional fluoride, especially if you live in an industrial area where the air contains more of it. Fluorides are used as rat poisoning and, in some areas, it's regularly added to the drinking water. Fluoride is nearly equally healthy and damaging for the human body. Too much of it can cause a slow change of the bone structure and changes in the thyroid gland as well as nerve damage. 8mg of fluoride a day will lead to skeletal changes. Fluorides are a by-product in aluminum production. The upper limit in drinking water is 1.5mg/l.

Iodine (I) Iodine is an important element for the proper functioning of the thyroid glands. A lack of iodine can lead to a pathogenic enlargement of the gland (known as goitre, sometimes spelled 'goiter').

Too much iodine is also damaging. Often, iodine is added to bread, and many people use iodinated salt. The recommended daily dose is no more than 0.15-0.18mg.

Iron (Fe) The human body needs iron to produce red blood cells. The muscular substance, myoglobin, also contains iron. Women chronically lack iron because of their menstrual bleeding. A lack of iron results in tiredness, cold hands and feet, brittle fingernails, exhaustion and sleeplessness. Too much iron can damage the organs where it's stored. Vitamin C encourages the absorption of iron. The upper limit in drinking water is 200ng/l.

Lead (Pb) We have mentioned already that even small doses of lead are detrimental for the human body. In embryos, infants and small children, brain development is significantly impacted, and in adults it affects the production of red blood cells. Lead also damages the functioning of the central nervous system. Pregnant women, babies and young children shouldn't take any food prepared with drinking water. The upper limit for lead in the European Directive for Drinking Water is zero.

Potassium (Ka) Potassium is very important for the body's water balance as it regulates the osmotic pressure of the cells. Potassium prevents an organism drying out. Top athletes prefer high-potassium food, such as bananas. Potassium is also important for the transmission of nerve signals and muscle contraction. A lack of potassium results in weak muscles, constipation and chronic fatigue. The recommended daily intake of 3000/4000mg is normally met by a healthy diet.

Magnesium (Mg) Magnesium is very important for the building of bone and muscle cells as well as for sinews. Osteoporosis and kidney stones are sometimes treated with magnesium. A lack of magnesium can cause leg cramps.

Natrium (Na) Natrium is needed for transporting water between cells.

Together with chlorine it forms sodium chloride, our cooking salt. When looking at the salt content of a mineral water please also note the chlorine content apart from the natrium content, as you take a lot of salt in with your daily diet. Upper limit: 50mg/l.

Silicate (Slo2) Silicates are useful in flushing out toxic substances. They're also involved in the building of bones, teeth and connective tissues.

Sulfate (SO4) Sulfate is a salt of sulfuric acid. Many chemical fertilizers and pesticides contain sulfates. Sulfate can increase the corrosion in water pipes. Too much sulfate can cause diarrhea. Minute quantities – even as low as 200mg/l – can interfere with the function of the colon. Please check the mineral water label whether it meets the EU Directive of an upper limit of 25mg/l.

Zinc (Zn) Zinc is a very important trace element as a building-block for DNA. A lack of zinc can be a cause of male infertility. Zinc creams are well-known for their healing powers. The whole immune system is boosted by zinc.

Our water is of different 'hardness' or 'softness', depending on the calcium content. Please see the table below for more information.

Concentration of CaCO3	Results in
0-75mg/l	soft water
75-150mg/l	medium soft water
150-300mg/l	hard water
Above 300mg/l	very hard water

Is water alive only because it sparkles?

More and more people get a soda machine for their household to avoid carrying and recycling the heavy glass or plastic bottles containing mineral water. Those machines supposedly turn your drinking water into a healthy, refreshing drink by adding carbon dioxide.

What happens? Some CO_2 is added to ordinary tap water. But it doesn't mean that you have now created mineral water. All the disadvantages of the tap water remain as you add only the metabolic waste product and preserving agent carbon dioxide which, in water, partially dissolves to carbonic acid, and wouldn't do anything to enhance your health. I'm sorry to disappoint you if you had hoped to have found a cheaper way to get mineral water. You also need to change the cartridges regularly to avoid contamination with germs.

I'm often asked what kind of water I use. I drink only spring water from a glass bottle. I either fill the bottle at the source or buy it in the supermarket. In any case, it's in a glass bottle and contains as few minerals as possible, because my wholemeal diet supplies me with enough minerals. This prevents an oversupply of minerals in the body.

The containers for making sparkling water need to be replaced regularly. And the cartridges are an additional piece of garbage for the landfill.

It's much better to order your supply of good mineral water with your online delivery of food. An alternative could be a filtering system for your tap water.

Water filters

There are many, many ways of filtering your tap water, but to do it is essential. Boiling only kills potential germs, but not the heavy metals.

There are many filtering systems available, and it may be difficult to make a good choice. Adding to the confusion is that they're all advertised as the best possible product. I have done a lot of research on water filters. The first device I bought was a normal table-top gadget with cartridges. Tea made with this filtered water looked and tasted differently. Unfortunately, I often forgot to change the cartridge and never knew whether the filtered-out harmful substances now re-entered the supposedly clean filtered water.

Please test the filtered water before you buy a filter. You'll be surprised how differently water can taste. It doesn't make sense to buy an expensive filter and you never drink the water because you don't like it or the tea tastes differently.

But I also discovered that this device didn't filter out the heavy metals I had wanted to get rid of. Calcium and magnesium were removed, but the cartridge also had the tendency to harbor germs. To prevent this, activated carbon or silver might be added which in turn gets into the water.

There is an activated carbon and granulate filter on the market, but I've never bought one. It does filter out chlorine and its components from the water but also develops many bacteria. An activated carbon-block filter removes a large amount of harmful substances from the water, together with asbestos fibers, chlorine, residues of medications, bacteria, pesticides and other small particles, but not minerals, nitrate and nitrites. The activated carbon membrane needs to be replaced every six months.

After my extensive research, I concluded that reverse osmosis is the most reliable way of removing heavy metals, pesticides, microorganisms, chlorine and its by-products, asbestos fibers, nitrate, nitrite and minerals from the water.

These devices have been developed in the US to desalinate sea water and are easily understandable. The tap water is pressed through a semi-porous membrane which lets only water molecules through. All other substances with molecules larger than water molecules are filtered out. Those substances are discarded by the rinsing process at the end.

If you decide to go for this device, please have it installed by a professional who also looks after the maintenance.

Water enhancement

You can filter out harmful substances from your drinking water but their electric vibration doesn't disappear.

The physicist Wolfgang Ludwig has evidenced how damaging these vibrations of harmful substances can be for our body. One should vitalize the drinking water to eliminate those negative vibration patterns.

Water has the ability to remember. Water has a memory – it stores information and can pass it on. Because of its unique structure water can bond time and again to form new water crystals. The most beautiful crystal formations can be found in healthy spring water.

Did you know that when you thaw a snowflake and then refreeze it, it will take on the same crystal structure as before?

When our drinking water is pure, healthy and alive, it can be optimally utilized by the organism. It can meet the requirement to be food stuff, a means to be alive. Pioneers researching the art of revitalizing water have been around for a long time. Just by observing nature, they recognized the flowing behavior of water and its healing properties.

Johann Grander and magnetic water information

The Austrian natural scientist Johann Grander is well known for vitalizing water. For over 20 years Grander experimented with magnetic plates and fields until he found water with a very high vibration frequency. His method of revitalizing water is based on a bio-technical procedure returning the lost information and energy back to the water. Magnetism causes high frequency vibrations of up to 100,000 hertz. This 'informed' water is pumped into chambers and normal water forced to flow over it. In a resonating process the flowing water is supplied with the information and vitalized. To obtain Grander-Water, there are several devices available which you can install in your water supply, but also larger devices for installation in ponds and swimming pools.

"Responsible people on this planet should have looked closer at nature and its creator as teachers, in which case we would now be on the right path with increased wealth and without environmental disasters."

JOHANN GRANDER

Wilfried Hacheney and his levitated water

The physicist Wilfried Hacheney (1924-2010) invented a patented procedure for vitalizing water. He assumed that we cannot judge drinking water by studying only its chemical composition but also by looking at its structure. A good parallel would be a diamond, as chemically the precious stone is nothing but graphite, but the structure makes it a completely different item.

Hacheney was particularly interested in water structure. He designed and built a container from stainless steel with a rotor inside which causes the water to accelerate and flow in a particular way. The water structure gets broken up into tiny droplets of up to 50 nanometers in size. With the changed structure, the water regains its original capacity to take up other substances and information. When you drink levitated water, you'll know instantly how detoxifying it is.

Hacheney calls this water levitated (from Latin: *levis* = light), as it favors processes opposing gravity.

Viktor Schauberger

Another well-known pioneer in vitalizing water was Viktor Schauberger (1885-1958). For years, he observed the flowing characteristics of water and developed a method to return its original structure to it. His son Walter (1914-1994) continued his father's work and developed a funnel for de-swirling, to break up and reorganize the cluster structure of tap water. It's a very simple experiment which you can try yourself. Take a bottle of water and empty it after having turned the bottle clockwise a few times. You'll see that the water flows out in a spiraling way and with increased speed. This spiraling flow can be produced by a special device installed into your tap. It also refines the cluster structure of the water. The water tastes 'softer' and is more able to meet its task as a transporting and dissolving agent in the human body.

Only the best: food containing lots of water

Plants are another miracle of nature and they offer the best substances we can give to our body: pure minerals, vitamins and trace elements. Plants are the only living beings able to transform sunlight into food by photosynthesis.

Vegetables – edible water

With the help of sunrays, plant cells abstract many organic minerals from the soil which, genetically, are perfectly compatible with the human body.

Inorganic minerals in plant *fluids* are different. They're a precious way to a healthy life. They also contain many secondary plant substances which can reduce the risk of cancer, catch free radicals and protect from infections. They also contribute to the blood flowing freely.

> TIP: the water contained in cauliflower, broccoli, peas, fennel, cucumber, cabbages, Swiss chard, carrots, peppers, leeks, beetroot, lettuces, celery, asparagus, spinach, tomatoes, zucchini, aubergines, artichokes and onions are valuable fluids and easily absorbed by the human body. The water content of these vegetables is between 82 and 95%

How to cook vegetables?

It's important to know how to prepare vegetables without destroying their valuable vitamins and minerals. It's recommended to prepare your meals only from fresh ingredients, not to keep leftovers for the next day or prepare food a day ahead. The longer a meal is kept, the more vitamins and other important substances evaporate. Only a few minutes after squeezing an orange for juice, it loses 50% of its vitamin contents. Vitamins also get destroyed by the cooking process. When you put a spoonful of honey in your tea, the valuable substances in the honey get destroyed by the heat.

Fresh, crisp salads are full of vitamins, but if you don't want to eat salads every day and don't like them much in the winter, you can prepare other healthy meals for yourself and your family – day in, day out.

The following methods of cooking and preparing vegetables are particularly gentle regarding vitamins and minerals.

Boiling You can cook vegetables and pulses completely immersed in water, but not for too long so not too many vitamins and valuable minerals evaporate. With soups, this is no problem as the dissolved substances are eaten with the broth. If you strain the food, you throw out valuable substances with the water. Try and use the liquids for other meals, soups and sauces.

Blanching This is a very short cooking process: you dip the vegetables briefly in boiling water and then plunge into ice water.

Steaming The vegetables are cooked in a steamer on top of a pot with boiling water. Steaming is also a gentle way of heating up a meal and better than by microwave. The look and taste of the vegetables are preserved. With longer cooking, the vital elements of the vegetables are dissolved in the water which can be reused.

Stewing This is a method suitable for vegetables not needing a longer cooking time. The food is given only very little water and the pot is closed with a tight lid to create a small water cycle: steam rises, condenses under the lid, and drips down – again and again, until the vegetables are cooked. The temperature should be low to prevent burning

The following vitamins are easily lost during cooking:

- B Vitamins: up to 45% loss
- Vitamin D: up to 30% loss
- Vitamin E: Up to 50% loss
- Folic acid: nearly 90% loss
- Vitamin C: 20-80% loss
- Biotin: up to 70% loss

Please don't cook, blanch, stew or boil any vegetables longer than necessary!

Food with a high water content

Secondary plant matter is responsible for the color, aroma and scent of a vegetable or fruit.

Primary plant matters are carbon hydrates, proteins and lipids.

International studies have shown that a healthy diet can reduce the risk of contracting cancer by up to 40%.

Artichokes

Artichokes have a beneficial effect on the liver, gall bladder and stomach. Bile production is stimulated and the liver can regenerate more efficiently. Artichokes also lower cholesterol and glucose levels. This is particularly important for diabetics. Artichokes help with rheumatism, gout, bladder and kidney complaints, diarrhea and excessive stomach acid. They contain calcium, potassium, magnesium, phosphorus, zinc and folic acid.

Asparagus

Asparagus flushes out toxins contained in food stuff and existing uric acid crystals from muscle tissue. Asparagus supports liver and lung function, boosts the kidneys' processes and is important for producing hormones. It contains a lot of iron, vitamin C, vitamin A, 'B' vitamins, calcium, phosphor, iodine, saponin and flavones. Green asparagus contains more minerals, vitamin C and carotenoids than white asparagus. While most people would benefit from its blood-cleansing effect, those with chronic kidney problems should avoid asparagus.

Aubergines

Aubergines contain 92% water. All nutrients are contained in the peel, so it's best to eat the whole fruit. They contain a lot of potassium, calcium, 'B' vitamins, phenol acids and bitter substances, which are beneficial for the liver. Aubergines are said to be helpful with rheumatism, sciatica, high cholesterol, kidney problems and diabetes. They dehydrate and promote the formation of new blood cells. Avoid aubergines if you have stomach ulcers.

Beetroot

Beetroot is highly regarded because of its high iron content. This stimulates the building of red blood cells and strengthens the vessels. Cell metabolism is increased which protects them from free radicals. Beetroot stimulates both bile flow and appetite. It deacidifies the body. Beetroot contains valuable amino acids, flavones, iodine, phosphor, protein, calcium, sugar, iron, copper, magnesium, pantothenic acid, folic acid, provitamin A, vitamins A, B and C, and potassium.

Broccoli

Contains a lot of carotene, vitamin C, vitamin E, 'B' vitamins, potassium, calcium, selenium, zinc, flavone and iron. Broccoli helps prevent cataracts.

The high carotene content also benefits the nerves and skin.

Cabbage

Cabbage lowers cholesterol levels and stops infections, while the roughage it contains is good for gut movement. Cabbage can prevent cancers and protects against heart attacks and strokes. A drink of cabbage juice is helpful with stomach ulcers and viral illness. Cabbage contains vitamin C, calcium, potassium, provitamin A, iron, copper and various 'B' vitamins, as well as indole which regulates the metabolism of estrogenic levels. Eaten daily, it can protect against breast cancer.

Carrots

Carrots contain a lot of alpha and beta-carotene, 'B' vitamins, folic acid, calcium, pectin, magnesium, phosphor and iron. The pectin content makes carrots highly digestible as it protects the mucus membranes in the stomach and gut. Beta-carotene is necessary for healthy eyesight, hair and skin. It's an important substance to protect cells from premature aging. When suffering from stress, night blindness, arteriosclerosis or diarrhea, a salad of raw carrots can be very beneficial.

Cauliflower

Cauliflower is high in vitamin C and contains potassium and few calories. It's suitable for a light diet as it's easily digestible.

Celery

Bulb celery is beneficially dehydrating and contains many volatile oils, resulting in a distinctive and pleasant taste. It contains vitamins E and B_6, folic acid, potassium and calcium.

Cucumber

The cucumber is an all-round champion! It contains many electrolytes and as a juice is highly suitable when exercising. It's dehydrating and stimulates the production of uric acid. It contains few calories as well as potassium, calcium and bitter substances which stimulate liver function. As they're very alkaline they support the heart function and lower cholesterol levels.

Fennel

Amazingly, fennel contains twice as much vitamin C as oranges. It contains menthol oil, anethole and fenchone – as well as iron, folic acid, vitamin E, beta-carotene, magnesium, potassium and calcium.

Garlic

Two–to-three cloves a day can drastically reduce the risk of arteriosclerosis. Garlic bulbs are powerful in deactivating germs, viruses, bacteria and other harmful substances. Garlic contains antioxidants and boosts the immune system. It can prevent cancer and heart attacks and lowers cholesterol levels. Garlic contains selenium, many vitamins and trace elements, and boosts blood circulation in the brain.

Kohlrabi

All cabbages contain high levels of vitamins C and K, provitamin A as well as calcium, potassium, magnesium and iron.

Kohlrabi also contains carbon hydrates, phosphor, folic acid and vitamins B_1, B_2 and B_6, all of which boost your immune system. The distinctive scent of kohlrabi when cooked is due to mustard oil which kills fungi and bacteria. It works well against infections of all kinds, as this oil boosts the building of white blood cells.

Leek

This allium plant contains the minerals potassium, iron and calcium; vitamins B_6, K and C; provitamin A, folic acid and volatile oils. Like all allium plants it has an antiseptic effect.

Lettuce

We're talking green salad leaves, containing high-grade protein as well as vitamin C, carotene, calcium, potassium, copper, folic acid, traces of zinc, manganese, selenium, iodine and chlorophyll, in addition to soporific substances. It's suggested that lettuce is good for alleviating sleep problems, stress and overstimulation.

Lettuce lowers blood pressure and uric acid levels. Green lettuce is recommended for those with diabetes, and it also lowers the risk of cancer, particularly stomach cancer. The risk of heart disease is reduced, too.

Despite its qualities, don't eat lettuce late at night because raw vegetables aren't easily digestible.

Onions

Onions are an old household remedy for earaches and illnesses of the respiratory tract. Onions protect from stomach cancer, heart disease and strokes. Volatile oils containing phosphor work as a natural antibiotic and antiseptic. Onions can kill bacteria, viruses and fungi, they flush water from the body and prevent blood clots. Our teeth, nails and bones are strengthened by the phosphor and calcium. Onions also contain many 'B' vitamins, vitamin C, potassium, iodine, selenium and the hormone-like prostaglandin A.

Peas

The good thing about peas is that they don't absorb many harmful substances from their environment as they're protected by the pod.

> TIP: dried peas should be soaked in water overnight. They contain a lot of phosphor, iron, phenolic acids and flavone.

Peas contain the vitamins B_1, B_2, B_3, C and E, as well as carotene, potassium, magnesium, a little zinc, lecithin and saponin.

Peppers

Most beneficial substances can be found in red peppers: provitamin A, vitamin E, beta-carotene, potassium, calcium, phosphor, magnesium, iron and twice as much vitamin C as in a lemon. Peppers are delicious eaten raw, which is best. They can boost skin circulation, strengthen the heart and blood vessels and improve eyesight. Peppers also boost the immune system and, with their capsaicin content, work as an aphrodisiac.

Potatoes

Gout, rheumatism and metabolic problems can be helped by a potato-based diet.

Potatoes can really help to keep you slim – as long as you don't fry them in fat. Their dehydrating potassium and trace elements boost the production of enzymes and make you feel full quickly. Potatoes contain a lot of starches, protein, magnesium, folic acid, vitamin C, phosphor, copper, zinc, cobalt and 'B' vitamins.

Swiss chard or mangold

Swiss chard contains very few calories and boasts many bio-active substances which protect against various illnesses.

This is very much an undervalued vegetable and we don't eat enough of it, despite it being a treasure trove of beneficial substances: potassium, calcium, magnesium, iron, vitamins B_1 and B_2, folic acid and a lot of vitamin C.

These substances reduce lipids in the blood, detoxify the gut, balance the digestive system and boost the immune system.

Spinach

Among other substances, spinach contains the hormone-like secretin which boosts the pancreas function. This leafy green vegetable is rich in beta-carotene, lutein, folic acid, calcium, magnesium, vitamins E and C, iodine, phosphor, iron and high-grade protein. It's very good for the prevention of cardiac problems and strokes. The carotene improves eyesight and the skin.

Tomatoes

My favorite! They're bursting with various beneficial phytol substances, such as terpene, flavone and carotene, as well as vitamins A, E and C. Tomatoes also contain important trace elements of zinc, nickel and cobalt – and, of course, iron, magnesium, calcium, 'B' vitamins, copper and phosphor.

Tomatoes help with blood production, protect against cancer, stimulate appetite, lower blood pressure, support the liver in detoxifying the body and cleanse the gut from putrid bacteria.

Zucchini

This vegetable contains a lot of beta-carotene, selenium, manganese, phosphor, potassium, calcium, folic acid, vitamin C and bitter substances. It's easily digestible and suitable for a light diet. It stimulates processes within the gut and dehydrates the organism. The health of both the liver and gall bladder are boosted, benefiting the kidneys and bladder. Carotene and selenium, also found in zucchini, are regarded as protective against cancer.

Water content in fruit

You can eat water! Many fruits have such a high water content that you can – nearly – do without additional drinks. To achieve this, you need to eat up to two kilograms of fruit and vegetables a day. If that is too much for you, you can always add some mineral water.

Watermelons, strawberries and grapes contain up to 95% water. In addition, this 'water' also contains trace elements of minerals and vitamins. Losing weight is made very easy if you eat an apple rather than just another sweet.

High-grade 'fruit-water' is contained in apples, pineapples, pears, strawberries, grapefruit, raspberries, currants, cherries, kiwi, rhubarb, tangerines, mangoes, melons, nectarines, oranges, papaya, peaches, plums, grapes and lemons

Our diet is constantly being checked and evaluated, and the latest scientific results confirm time and again that many heart problems, strokes and metabolic illnesses can be avoided by adopting a better diet.

To change your diet, just gradually introduce more fruit and vegetables into your daily menu plan. Take time to test out delicious new recipes and try to do without processed food and ready meals. If you don't have much time for cooking, then it's always much better to eat a banana or a tomato sandwich with chives rather than put something into the microwave. It's the best 'fast food' ever!

An apple a day really does keep the doctor away!

Apples

This is a real 'power fruit', and you should only wash it, not peel it. Apples contain about 300 different bio-substances, such as pectin, vitamins C and B, potassium, calcium, phosphor, iron, natrium, fruit sugar, tanning agents and organic acids. Pectin lowers cholesterol. An apple refreshes in the morning and helps you sleep at night. It helps the body to stop diarrhea, soothes itching, neutralizes toxins in the gut and fights infections.

The pectin in ripe apples bonds with harmful substances in the gut and helps to digest them.

Cherries

Darker varieties contain a lot of valuable substances, such as flavones, potassium, iron, magnesium, silicic acid, phosphor, vitamin C, carotene and the vitamins B_1, B_2 and B_3. Silicic acid nourishes bones, teeth and nails. Cherries stimulate digestion and benefit the heart and the cardiac system, liver and kidneys by dehydrating the body of excess fluid.

Grapes

Grapes are rich in vitamin C, 'B' vitamins, fructose, pectin, ellagic acid, potassium and various anti-germ substances. Grapes detoxify and purge and help digesting lipids.

> TIP: grapes are often treated with various substances during growing, so please wash them carefully before eating.

Following inflammation of the liver, grapes support its regeneration. Bladder and kidney problems are helped as grapes build blood. Grapes protect from arteriosclerosis, strengthen the heart and reduce uric acid.

Grapefruit

The grapefruit is known as the 'fat-absorber' on the breakfast table. It's high in potassium, vitamin C and fruit acids, has a dehydrating effect, purges, thins the blood and prevents the formation of crystals in the body.

Grapefruits are recommended for low blood pressure as well as increased levels of uric acid and cholesterol.

Kiwis

This fruit, originating in New Zealand, is high in vitamin C (it contains three times as much as citrus fruits) which is one reason why it's popular for fighting infections and exhaustion. Kiwis firm up connective tissues and blood vessels, cleanse the blood, increase urine production and help to digest proteins.

Lemons

Familiar advice when a cold is in the offing is: have a hot lemon! The high content of vitamin C makes lemons a popular household remedy. Lemons can lower a high temperature, kill bacteria, flush out toxins and waste products from the gut, and lemon peel helps with skin complaints. Use only organic lemons and slice the whole fruit.

Mangoes

Mangoes are very good for people with a sensitive stomach as they have a beneficial impact on the digestive system. Their high iron content promotes blood-building processes. Mangoes stimulate the regeneration of the nervous and glandular systems, and the brain. With their high content of beta-carotene, they benefit mucus membranes. They prevent dry eyes, and the immune system is boosted by their properties. Mangoes are also rich in 'B' vitamins, vitamin E, iron and flavones.

Melons

Attention! Because melons stimulate the gall bladder, too much of it can cause diarrhea.

Especially in the summer, melons are perfect to quench the thirst as they're more than 90% water. Melons dehydrate the body and, as a consequence, flush the kidneys out and get rid of excess salt and uric acid.

They cleanse the blood and thin it and stimulate the digestive system. Melons contain valuable fruit acids, magnesium, phosphor, calcium, iron and vitamins A and C.

Oranges

Oranges are high in beta-carotene, vitamins C and E and the 'B' group, potassium, phosphor, bio-flavonoids, folic acid, selenium, calcium and lutein. They boost the immune system and help to prevent heart disease and strokes. Oranges reduce harmful LDL-cholesterols and can help combat varicose veins as this particular fruit improves blood-flow through the capillaries (smaller blood vessels).

Papayas

I would put the papaya first, before all other exotic fruit, as it's rich in papain, an important enzyme for processing proteins. When feeling uncomfortable after a meal and fearing digestive problems, eat a fresh papaya, as it will stimulate metabolism. The gut is cleansed from the protein residues still in the body; they're broken up and discarded faster. Papayas are rich in beta-carotene, provitamin A, vitamin C, calcium, potassium, iron, magnesium, carotenoids, flavonoids, vitamins B_1, B_2, B_3, vitamin E and niacin.

Papayas help those who are overweight, or have high acidity or blood pressure, constipation, varicose veins, infections or arteriosclerosis.

Peaches and nectarines

Because of their high zinc content, these fruits can improve semen production in men. They also contain vitamins A, B and C, magnesium, calcium, potassium, iron, natrium, flavones and beta-carotene. They boost the immune system and dehydrate as they improve kidney function.

Pears

Pears contain a lot of fructose and make you feel full quickly. They increase gut movement and help digestion. They're high in potassium and dehydrate the organism. Tanning agents found in pears can have a soothing effect on inflammations of the stomach and gut. Pears are also rich in vitamin C, magnesium, calcium, phosphor, zinc, copper, iodine, fructose and carotene. They boost the kidneys and protect the body from too much acid.

Pineapple

To get all the good stuff from pineapples you should eat only fresh ones. Pineapples boost the processing of lipids with the enzyme bromalin. This helps with losing weight and breaking down animal protein. Pineapples contain magnesium, phosphor, potassium, manganese, zinc, iodine, vitamin C and carotene. They stimulate the appetite, cleanse the blood and also help with infections.

Plums

Whether dried or fresh, plums contain a lot of iron and speed up digestion. Toxins are expelled from the gut more quickly, and the production of stomach acid is increased.

> TIP: when traveling, the digestive system often doesn't work well. Take some dried plums to snack on regularly, and it will soon be okay again.

Plums contain carotene, copper, zinc, potassium, natrium, phosphor, calcium, anthocyanins and vitamins B_1 and B_2. They're also said to guard against cancers.

Raspberries

Raspberries contain significant amounts of potassium, magnesium, iron, phosphor, pectin, tanning agents, flavones and salicylic acid. They support the detoxification process of the liver, regenerate the mucus membranes in the gut and support bone formation. They're important for all nerve processes and the brain.

Rhubarb

Rhubarb contains a lot of minerals, but you need to exercise some caution: not too much of it, and never eat it raw, as rhubarb contains oxalic acid which, in combination with calcium, can cause kidney stones. If you suffer from gout, rheumatism or arthritis – do without rhubarb. It contains calcium, magnesium, iron, phosphor, iodine and volatile oils, glycosides and pectin as well as lemon and apple acids. Their vitamin content is negligible. Rhubarb has a blood-cleansing and detoxifying effect on the body.

Redcurrants and blackcurrants

These tasty berries are a vitamin C powerhouse! More than twice your recommended daily allowance is contained in just 100g of currants. They also contain many 'B' vitamins, flavones, phosphor, calcium and several other minerals. The high vitamin C content helps to support the immune system and maintain blood vessels' elasticity. The currants' coloring agents benefit the metabolism of the brain, as well as gland and cell functions. In case of diarrhea, currant juice has a detoxifying and cleansing effect.

Strawberries

Strawberries contain more vitamin C than lemons! This little fruit boasts more than 300 different valuable substances, such as pectin, flavones, potassium, calcium, phosphor, iron, natrium, volatile oils and tanning agents. Thus, they improve digestion, speed up healing processes and prevent muscle cramps.

Tangerines

Tangerines contain provitamin A, vitamin C, minerals and a lot of fructose. They boost the immune system because of their high vitamin C content. Tangerines also improve the appetite and quench thirst.

> TIP: if you want to make a change from taking bottled water everywhere, just put some tangerines in your handbag. They're easy to peel and quench thirst most wonderfully.

Vitamins and what they do

We have now learned about the vitamin and mineral content in the most important vegetables and fruit. In the following, you'll find an overview of what these valuable substances actually do for your body.

It's a good idea to get to know your body better – and to listen to it. It will tell you exactly and clearly what is good for you and what's not. Start with a detoxification and concentrate on your inner self, to be sensitive to what it tells you. Your good health will be your best reward.

Vitamin A

This vitamin is responsible for the maintenance of mucus membranes and the formation of rhodopsin, which helps to maintain your eyesight. It regenerates cells and is important for fertility.

Vitamin B1 (thiamine)

This is the vitamin for the nerves. It boosts concentration and is important for circulation.

Vitamin B2 (riboflavin)

An important vitamin for healthy skin and hair, it's also needed for cell growth and supports eyesight.

Vitamin B3 (niacin)

This vitamin is important for metabolism. It can reduce cholesterol levels and has a stimulating effect on circulation.

Vitamin B5 (pantothenic acid)

Vitamin B_5 is also called the anti-stress vitamin as it helps with depression and anxiety. It boosts concentration and prevents the premature aging of the skin.

Vitamin B6 (pyridoxine)

This vitamin is important for the nervous system and the breakdown of proteins. If we don't get enough of it, symptoms may include cardiac problems, weak muscles, nervousness and mood swings.

You can easily avoid a bad diet because there are so many alternatives to provide your body with enough vitamins and minerals.

Vitamin B12 (cobalamin)

… is important for cell growth and cell division. Metabolism in the brain and nervous system are also influenced by vitamin B_{12}, which contributes to the formation of red blood cells.

Folic acid

Folic acid is important for protein metabolism, the production of red blood cells and cell growth. It contributes to the building of DNA and RNA. During pregnancy, folic acid is particularly important for the development of the foetus.

Vitamin C

Very important for the immune system. It strengthens connective tissue and the blood vessels and is also known to effectively break down lipids.

Vitamin E

… supports circulation and protects from arteriosclerosis. It defers the aging process of the skin cells and guards against free radicals.

Vitamin K

This vitamin helps with the coagulation of the blood and contributes to building bone mass.

Secondary plant matter

These precious, bio-active substances are responsible for the beautiful colors of plants, their aroma and scent. They make tomatoes red and grapefruit bitter. In more than 20 years of research, over 30,000 substances have been discovered, of which only 10,000 are in plant-based food. Time and again, scientists have concluded that people with a vegetarian diet or who daily eat a lot of fruit and vegetables are at less risk of cancer and heart diseases. There are signs that secondary plant substances can actually block cancer, boost the immune system and catch free radicals in the body.

High-grade water from plants - with their important vitamins and minerals - is sufficient to stay healthy and stimulate the fantastic self-healing capacity of the human body. Let's look at the most important of these magic substances.

Carotenoids

They're contained in yellow, orange and red vegetables, fruit and some green vegetables. Carotenoids are said to block the development of cancer and boost the immune system.

Flavonoids

Are contained in most plant-based food and protect from free radicals. They also have an anti-inflammatory effect.

Glucosinolates

These aromatic substances can be found in cress, Brussels sprouts, horseradish and mustard. They reduce cholesterol, have an antioxidizing effect and prevent infections. They're also antibacterial.

Phenolic acids

These have an anti-inflammatory effect, normalise blood pressure and can be found in apples, broccoli, carrots, grapes and onions.

Phyto-estrogens

These can block cancerous development and fight free radicals. Contained in barley, wheat, linseed and soybeans. Helpful for the building of bone mass.

Phytosteroles

These can have an anti-cancer effect and reduce cholesterol levels. Contained in sunflower seeds and sesame seeds.

Saponines

This is a rather bitter substance and could help to protect from fungal infections. Stimulates the immune system.

Sulphides

…boost the immune system and balance blood pressure - contained in broccoli, kale, linseed and onions.

Terpenes

…have a cancer-blocking effect and are contained in fennel, kale, carrots, onions, garlic, celery, lemons and oranges.

The myth of cow's milk

Cow's milk is the mother's milk for calves. Its task is to make calves grow as quickly as possible to reach their reproductive age and to supply them with important nutrients during the growth period. But are you a calf? And do our babies need to be fertile and ready for reproduction within 24 months?

It's not surprising that these days we're dealing with allergies much more often. Cow's milk contains substances that the human body finds difficult to digest. No other animal would dream of drinking the milk from a different creature, because mother's milk is always perfectly geared to bring up one's own species – just as human mother's milk is perfectly adapted for human babies. Would you drink milk from a kangaroo?

Once the calf has grown, it never drinks milk again. And you? Do you drink your mother's milk once you're grown up?

Many physicians have concluded that milk often causes allergies and other illnesses. Cow's milk produces mucus, and this mucus clings to the organs and to our respiratory system; it makes digestion more difficult. Bronchitis, sinusitis, ear infections and headaches can all be related to the consumption of cow's milk. Some kinds of cheese contain a protein which causes migraine.

The human body needs enzymes to process and digest two components of dairy products: casein and lactose. Casein is broken down by the enzyme rennin. After the age of four, the human body no longer produces rennin.

Cow's milk contains about 300 times more casein than human milk. Cows need casein to build their large bones. In human stomachs, casein curdles and turns into indigestible, tough mucus clusters. The cow's four stomachs have no problem with that, but the human stomach finds it difficult to get rid of all this mucus. The cell walls of the gut get clotted, and villi in the small intestine cannot extract the nutrients from the rest of the diet. About 98% of people have a lactose intolerance, and to be able to digest milk, we're given more medication – a fatal cycle!

Furthermore, the calcium contained in cow's milk – one reason drinking milk is often recommended – can only partly be digested by the human body, because for this process it needs magnesium, which isn't contained in cow's milk. A lot of calcium in cow's milk doesn't mean a lot of calcium for the human body. A diet rich in animal protein often leads to a lack of calcium. This sheds a different light on the bone disease, osteoporosis.

The answer to this is that with a meat-free diet you don't need so much calcium, because it's contained naturally in many vegetables, fruit and nuts. Almonds, sesame seeds and soya products contain calcium which is digested easily by the human body.

100g of almonds contains twice as much calcium as 100ml of cow's milk, sesame seeds hold six times as much!

Water and salt – a love story

"Salt bonds with water," my grandmother used to say, when I, again – without having tasted my food – simply took the salt cellar and sprinkled the little white crystals all over my meal. I knew what she meant, but I didn't really understand it then. Today I know about the problems resulting from too much salt in the body. On top of it all, we use natrium chloride as table salt, which is capable of storing an enormous amount of water in the body. And it's much more difficult to flush out.

Table salt

Table salt has been industrially cleaned, and all valuable minerals are extracted in the process. It's then bleached and given a synthetic flowing agent. The end result is not the high-grade salt necessary for cell-building in the human body.

On the contrary, our bodies need salt which is pure, untreated and contains all the essential trace elements and minerals. Before I changed my diet, I took in 6g of salt daily, but the human body only needs about 0.2g. Anything more, and it will be stored somewhere in the organism because

> Too much salt can do as much damage as too little. It's very important that you choose the right kind of salt.

it can't be flushed out easily. The average person daily consumes between 7g and 9g of salt. As processed food, such as sausages and crisps, contains additional amounts of salt, we don't really know anymore how much salt we consume daily. One consequence could be a large tummy which people think is just fat. But maybe it's just water stored in the connective tissue?

Crystal salt

The kinds of salt available widely – such as cooking salt, stone salt and sea salt – are all crystal salts, as their structure is crystalline, but their quality varies.

You've probably come across so-called 'Himalayan Crystal Salt'. In my view, it's a good choice and preferable to ordinary table salt.

Himalayan salt is natural and has maintained its extraordinary crystalline structure. Crystal salt has been exposed to enormous pressure over the millennia which helped to develop a most perfect crystalline structure.

> Apart from water, salt is a very important building-block for the human body. The more natural and pure it is, the better for us.

In this pure crystal salt, you find elements also contained in the human body, apart from many other needed minerals and trace elements. Himalayan salt is pale pink and is mined by hand. This, of course, is costly, but it is worth it because you won't use as much salt as before. Once the body has got used to this high-quality salt there is no urge anymore to add more salt to the food on your plate.

Sea salt

Sea salt is produced in salt lakes near the sea. The artificial pools are filled with sea water, and with the help of sun and wind the water evaporates, leaving the sea salt behind. You find saline plants on the shores of Portugal, Spain, France and many other places. After being collected, the sea salt is often bleached and mixed with a flowing agent. Precious minerals and trace elements get lost. Bio-sea salt, available in health-food shops, has not undergone this process and still contains the natural minerals and trace elements. In biologically managed salt plants, the water quality is also strictly controlled. Only this guarantees a high-grade sea salt.

Stone salt

This salt is mined from residues of evaporated, older, underground salt-water bodies. It's blasted-off in salt mines and then undergoes various processes to leave a high-quality table salt. But it's often bleached and mixed with flowing agents. This process means that many minerals and trace elements are eliminated. Untreated stone salt looks grey and 'dirty' but contains many important substances.

Saline salt

Salt stored underground is also called saline salt. It's mined by running hot water over it to dissolve it to create a saline solution, which is then pumped into large basins for the water to evaporate. This salt is treated chemically, meaning that valuable substances are lost. It's recommended to only use ecologically sound products to guarantee the necessary minerals and trace elements for the human body.

The beauty of water

Why is water capable of healing? The Japanese scientist, Masaru Emoto, came to the following answer to this question: "Water heals the human body because it returns the soul to its natural balance of vibrations."

Since the Eighties, Masaru Emoto has taken photos of various water samples from rivers, lakes, brooks, springs and taps from all over the world. His book, *The Message of Water*, enhanced our view of water and enabled us to not just consider it simply as two chemical ingredients – two parts oxygen and one part hydrogen. In his photos of water crystals, we recognize clearly that water is the source of all life.

Emoto's images speak for themselves, and we begin to understand why certain springs, such as in Lourdes, have healing powers. Emoto managed to take photos of breathtakingly beautiful water crystals to show that water is an ingenious carrier of vibrations. But his experiments went further: he played music to the water, and the water structure changed depending on the kind of music.

Classical music produces the most beautiful crystals, while certain pop or techno music can't bring the water to form crystals at all. For years, music therapy has been supportive in work with disabled children – with a healing effect. Encouraged by the success of his musical experiments, Emoto went a step further. He wrote various words and phrases on pieces of paper and stuck them on glasses filled with water. To the amazement of all witnesses, here, too, different crystals formed, depending on what was written on the labels. The vibration of the words was transferred to the water and the molecules formed different cluster structures.

> TIP: inspired by Emoto's work and by my own experience of how words and sounds can influence the soul, I developed the drinking glass series, *Water-Balance,* for daily use. Together with the renowned glass factory Spiegelau, we have created an extraordinary series of drinking glasses. They represent the Chinese philosophy of feng-shui on the one hand, and Western spiritual heritage on the other. We offer drinking glasses with the engravings of the words *Love, Joy, Harmony, Happiness, Thank you,* and *Light,* as well as with the Asian signs for *Love, Luck, Lust, Hope, Peace* and *Thanks.* These words and signs possess, according to Emoto, a strong power to load drinking water with their positive impact. The enriched water can encourage new energies in the human body and restore a healthy balance.

With his fascinating experiments and the impressive photos of water crystals, Emoto showed that words and prayers can be transferred to water. Some words are like arrows. You'll probably never forget certain sets of words. The power of the word can't be overestimated. If you hear, time and again, "You make me ill!", it's only a question of time until you experience the consequences. If you hear many loving and positive words, you'll always feel good. The same applies to water: it expresses word vibrations by forming beautiful crystals.

Water is an important carrier of information – and we consist of more than 70% water! You can imagine the effect negative or positive words can have. Our cell water is being 'coded' in the negative or positive direction. Prayers spoken over water give it a unique crystalline structure which is available to all participants as vibrations.

Water can also be changed when it's poured from one vessel into another. In all cultures and religions, pure water has always been kept in special jugs made from mountain crystal – in veneration to the precious gift of nature.

How to save precious water

- Collect rainwater in a butt under the gutters for watering your garden. It's environmentally friendly and reduces your water bill.

- Repair leaks in the water system quickly.

- Don't wash-up under running water – do it in the sink.

- When washing your car, please use as little water as possible. Also, when it comes to adding a cleaning agent, use as little as possible – you'll use less water to rinse it off.

- Only run the washing machine and dishwasher when they're fully loaded.

- Turn off the tap when cleaning your teeth.

- Install a water-saving device in the toilet cistern.

- Buy fruit and vegetables grown locally because of the transport involved in getting them to you. Importing them from far-away countries means extensive water-use there – which could mean it's not then available for the rest of the population.

Acknowledgments

All my life I have been lucky to meet very special people who gave my path a better, more important direction. They reminded me to listen to the call of my soul or simply embraced me lovingly. Most of all, I'm grateful to my husband Pierre Franckh, my soulmate, who supports me in everything I do. My daughter Julia is my best teacher, because she has shown me what unconditional love is.

Thank you, my friends, who have been with me for all these years.

I dedicate this book to all nature lovers and water creatures.

Michaela Merten

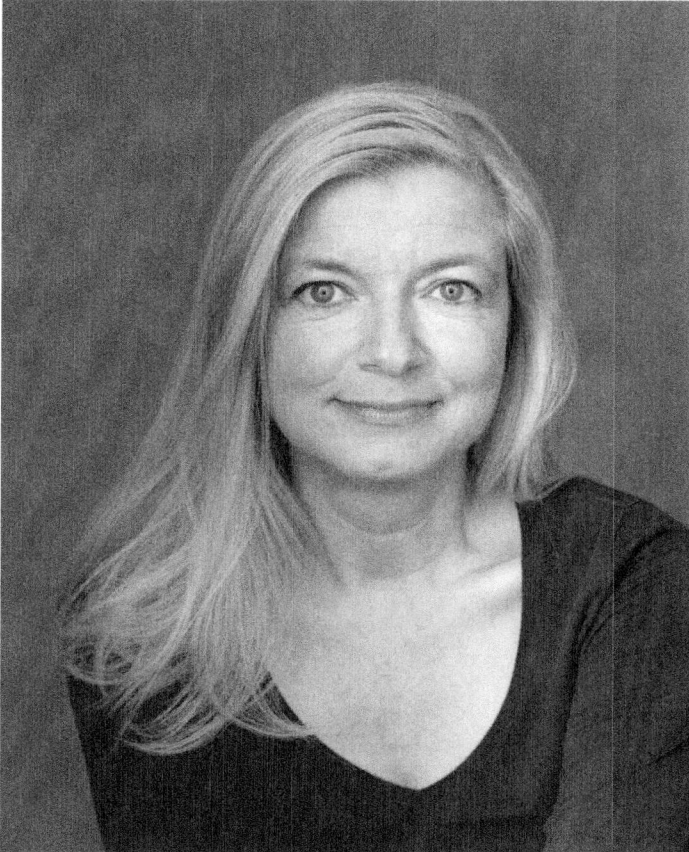

The bestselling author and keynote speaker Michaela Merten has been a fixture in film and TV for more than 30 years. As an actress, she starred in many national and international film productions. She attributes her success at least partly to being a success coach and author on happiness, mindfulness & meditation and wellbeing.

An expert on water and its benefits, her book, 'Water - the key to beauty and health', entered the bestseller lists in Germany soon after publication, and many other bestselling books on personal development followed. Her most popular books are published in English as well as German.

She is an ambassador for the Water Foundation and also provided a testimonial to the FIFA World Cup Beckenbauer Project in 2006.

For many years she has been working as a keynote speaker, creative consultant, motivational coach and a well-known coach for business leaders and celebrities.

Together with her husband and frequent co-author, Pierre Franckh – an international bestselling writer in his own right – they have published more than 40 titles, selling about 3.5 million copies in Germany alone. She also lectures, teaches and leads seminars and retreats in five countries.

Together, Michaela and Pierre founded Happiness House, an online academy and community for personal development.

Her coaching and consulting includes:

- How to achieve authentic happiness

- How to find the purpose of your life

- How to handle setbacks and defeats successfully

- How to best exploit your potential

- Your path to personal success

- Meditation as a path for inner peace

- How to turn your life into a personal masterpiece

www.happiness-house.de

www.Michaela-Merten.com

For further information please send email to:

contact@michaela-merten.com

Bibliography

Amthor, Silke: *Aquafitness*, Südwest Verlag
ISBN 3-517-065-57-9, 2002

Andersson, Michael: *Heilen mit Wasser*
Dr. Werner Jopp Verlag
ISBN 3-926955-78-3, 1993

Emoto, Masaru: *Die Botschaft des Wassers*

Bankhofer, Hademar:
Gesundheit aus der Badewanne
Delphin Verlag GmbH,
ISBN 3-7735-5208-4, 1984

Beigel-Guhl, Karen und Brinckman Andreas: *Wasser Gymnastik*
-3, 2001

Batmanghelidj, Fereydoon Dr. med.:
Man's Cry for Water: You are not sick, you are thirsty
Global Health Solutions
ISBN 978-0970245885

Batmanghelidj, Fereydoon Dr. med.:
Bantam Books
Man's Cry for Water: A Revolutionary Way to Prevent Illness and Restore Good Health
Tagman Press
ISBN 978-0953092161

Dalla Via, Gudrun:
Lichtwässer und ihre Heilkräfte
AT Verlag, Aarau, Schweiz
ISBN 3-85502-909-1, 2003

Dargatz, Thorsten und Röwekamp, Andrea:
Aqua Fitness
Copress Sport
ISBN 3-7679-1041-1, 2010

Diamond, Harvey und Marilyn: *Fit for Life I*
Bantam Books
ISBN 978-0553815887

Diamond Harvey und Marilyn: *Fit for Life II*
Bantam |Books
ISBN 978-0553175820

Emoto, Masaru: *Die Antwort des Wassers*
KOHA-Verlag
ISBN 3-929512-93-9, 2002

Emoto, Masaru:
Die Antwort des Wassers, Band 2
KOHA-Verlag
ISBN 3-929512-98-X, 2003

Exel, Wolfgang Dr. med. und Rohrer Karin: *Wasser heilt!*
Kneipp Verlag
ISBN 3-902191-05-8, 2002

Geisler, Linus Prof. Dr. med.:
Natürlich heilen mit Wasser
Naumann & Göbel Verlagsgesellschaft mbH
ISBN 3-625-10786-4

Geiss, Heide Marie Karin:
Kraftquelle Wasser
Trautwein Ratgeber Edition,
Compact Verlag München
ISBN 3-8174-5335-3, 2000

Hacheney, Friedrich: *Levitiertes Wasser*
Äquadukt Dingfelder Verlag
ISBN 3-926253-42-8, 1994

Hechtl, Christian und Oliver:
Wasser mit natürlich gelöstem Sauerstoff
ISBN 3-935585-31-4, 2001

Hechtl, Christian Prof. of Engg., Dr.-Ing.:
Gesundes Wasser ist nicht nur zum
Trinken da
ISBN 3-935585-00-4, 2001

Hendel, Barbara Dr. med., Ferreira, Peter:
Wasser & Salz
INA- Verlags GmbH
ISBN 3-000082-33-6, 2003

Hendel, Barbara Dr. med: *Wasser vom Reinsten*
Ina Verlags GmbH
ISBN 3-9808408-1-6, 2003

Heßmann-Kosaris, Anita:
Wasser ist die beste Medizin
Midena Verlag
ISBN 3-310-00247-0, 1998

Honauer, Urs: *Wasser – die geheimnisvolle*
Energie
Irisiana bei Heinrich Hugendubel Verlag
ISBN 3-89631-240-5, 1998

Hutzl-Ronge, Barbara:
Quellgöttinnen, Flussheilige,
Meerfrauen
Verlag Frauenoffensive

ISBN 3-88104-345-4, 2002

Katalyse e.V. Herausgeber:
Das Wasser-Buch,
Verlag Kiepenheuer & Witsch, Köln
ISBN 3-462020-37-4, 1990

Kaltenthaler, Birgit:
Powerdrink Sauerstoffwasser
Midena Verlag
ISBN 3-310006-94-8, 2002

Krahl Gisela und Riepe, Andrea:
Wonnestunden
Rowohlt Verlag GmbH
ISBN 3-805204-97-3, 1990

Kraus, Michael: *Ätherische Öle*
Verlag Simon & Wahl
ISBN 3-923330-16-2, 1991

Kronberger, Hans und Lattacher, Siegbert:
Auf der Spur des Wasserrätsels
Uranus Verlagsgesellschaft m.b.H.
ISBN 3-901626-01-8, 2001

Kröll, Thomas: *Die Wasserapotheke,*
Mosaik bei Wilhelm Goldmann Verlag
ISBN 3-442-16191-6, 1999

Moll, Karl und Spiller, Wolfgang:
Schachmatt den Allergien
Schnitzer Verlag
ISBN 3-922894-54-2, 1995

Oberbeil, Klaus: *Lebenselixier Wasser*
Südwest Verlag
ISBN 3-517-06693-1, 2003

Pittroff, Uschka und Niemann,
Christina und Regelin,
Petra: *Wellness,*
Gräfe und Unzer Verlag GmbH

Rhyner, Hans H.:
*Gesund leben, sanft heilen mit
Ayurveda*
Königsfurth-Urania Verlags AG
ISBN 3-908646-89-8, 2000

Ryrie, Charlie: *Heilende Energie
des Wassers*
Königsfurth-Urania Verlags AG
ISBN 3-908652-01-4, 1999

Seifen, Martina: *Die große
Farbdiät*
Verlagsgruppe Lübbe
Ehrenwirthlife
ISBN 3-431-04055-1, 2003

Walterskirchen, Helene: aqua
wellness
Ariston Verlag
ISBN 3-7205-2005-6, 1998

Zacker, Christina: *Vitalkur für den
Körper*
Wilhelm Heyne Verlag
ISBN 3-453-14801-0, 1999

Cellular Phone Task Force
The Work Of Leif Salford
http://www.cellphonetaskforce.
org/?page_id=579

Printed in Great Britain
by Amazon